Breakouts and Babies

7 Natural Ways To Get Rid Of Acne During Pregnancy

By Angela Knight

I0415614

Table of Contents

Introduction

Hormones - The Number 1 Cause Of Pregnancy Acne

It isn't just an old wives' tale; it's really true. A woman can look ravishing during pregnancy. Well, make that some women. Indeed, while pregnancy can leave some lucky ladies looking luscious, for others, all that extra hormonal activity can have the opposite effect, causing a variety of pregnancy skin problems. Hands down, acne is the No. 1 skin problem to hit women during pregnancy, but there are also a variety of bumps and rashes and discolorations that occur as well, most of them due to hormone activity.

Pregnancy can trigger acne or make existing adult acne worse. Higher levels of hormones called androgens are at least partly responsible for pregnancy breakouts because they can prompt the sebaceous glands in your skin to get bigger and boost production of an oily substance called sebum. This extra sebum, combined with the shed skin cells that line your hair follicles, blocks your pores, creating an environment in which bacteria can rapidly multiply. All this can eventually lead to the inflammation and skin eruptions of acne. Acne can vary in severity for each woman and may just be an early pregnancy thing, or may persist throughout your pregnancy.

Pregnancy acne is very unpredictable; some women who have battled acne before becoming pregnant may find that their acne improves, and others who have never had acne find that they have the most problems. If you do not develop acne during the first trimester, it's unlikely you'll have breakouts that are out of the ordinary during the second or third trimesters. Fortunately, the acne subsides once hormone levels return to normal. For women who typically have clear skin, acne usually disappears sometime after delivery, although it may last longer if the mother is breastfeeding.

The Top 5 Contributory Factors

Whilst hormonal imbalances are understood to be the main cause of acne during pregnancy, there are 5 other contributory factors:

1. Fluid retention: the increased levels of hormone in the body make it hold on to more fluid than normal. Retention of body fluid can contribute to acne breakouts due to the increased level of toxins contained in these fluids.

2. Dietary modifications: during pregnancy, it is very common among women to experience sudden hunger pangs. They are therefore tempted to consume fast foods that are usually oily and greasy. A diet that encourages or helps your acne to thrive is, however, something that you can do plenty about. Cutting out (or just cutting back on) sugar and refined grains can do wonders for your skin (opt for whole grains instead). Also, unhealthy fats (aka the saturated fats found in fried foods and many baked goods) can aggravate acne, so replace these with skin-boosting healthy fats like avocado, salmon, walnuts, and almonds. More skin friendly foods: colourful fresh fruits and vegetables and, believe it or not, small amounts of dark chocolate (the darker the better). Just eat in moderation!

3. Genetic characteristic: If your parents, or their parents, suffered from acne, then the chances that you will too are much higher, and unfortunately there is not a great deal that you can do about it.

4. Stress: Pregnant women are often under a great deal of stress, both physically and mentally, and this only serves to compound the problem. At times when the body is under strain or having to work excessively hard, the liver is incapable of dealing effectively with excess and spent hormones, and this is the reason that acne tends to flare up in times of stress.

5. Medicines: Pregnancy medications can sometimes cause side effects on the skin, resulting in acne breakouts. These acne breakouts can be more painful and itchy than normal.

Five Acne Myths

1. "Acne is caused by having dirty skin and poor hygiene."

Most of the biological reactions that trigger acne occur beneath the skin, not on the surface of the skin. Therefore, how clean your skin is will have little to no effect on your acne. You should wash your face twice a day. More frequent washing will make no difference to your acne. Don't be tempted to scrub your acne away. It won't work, and you'll end up stripping your skin of its natural moisture, which in turn will cause your oil glands to go into overdrive trying to replenish what you've removed.

2. "Squeezing blackheads, whiteheads and spots is the best way to get rid of acne."

As tempted as you might be. As your mother always warned you (and this time she's right), these tactics will only make acne last longer and can cause scars. It will encourage the transfer of dirt and oils into the wounds that you have irritated or opened with your actions, and cause deeper (and often more painful) acne lesions which are far more likely to cause scarring. Do not be tempted to squeeze blackheads or whiteheads that have formed as a result of your acne for exactly the same reasons.

3. "Sexual activity can influence acne."

Having sex or masturbating will not make acne any worse or any better. End of story!

4. "Sunbathing, sunbeds and sunlamps help improve the symptoms of acne."

There is no conclusive evidence that prolonged exposure to sunlight or using sunbeds or sunlamps can improve acne. Many medicines used to treat acne (including those that are safe to use during pregnancy) can make you more prone to sunburn. And while the sun may help dry out your acne lesions, that doesn't come without a price. Too much sun not only increases your risk of skin cancer and causes early aging of the skin, it can also bring on other blotches during pregnancy. Whenever you're going to be outside, use sunscreen of at least SPF 15 — and make that an oil-free one.

5. "Acne is infectious."

You cannot pass acne on to other people and it is not infectious. Fact!

Getting Rid of Pregnancy Acne: The Bottom Line

The skin is a complex and highly dynamic 'cover' for your body, one that is literally changing every second of the day as skin cells die, only to be replaced by new ones in a permanently revolving cycle of old life being rejuvenated by new. Most importantly, your skin reflects your general state of health, and protects you against the invasion of foreign infections and toxins. It also allows the body to pass the toxins that inevitably congregate inside it to be passed to the outside safely and efficiently. So, your skin is definitely worthy of a great deal of care and attention.

However, no matter how much care and attention you lavish upon your skin, it is virtually impossible to entirely prevent the onset of acne if you are predisposed to the condition through pregnancy. Furthermore, whatever you put on your skin moves into your body, by way of the bloodstream; so topical medications always have the potential to harm your baby. In general, you should avoid all medications you don't absolutely need during pregnancy, including seemingly harmless over-the-counter acne medications and chemical spot treatments. Let's take a closer look at the 3 most popular acne medications:

1. Accutane: This is a prescription medication that is taken orally to treat acne. The generic name for Accutane is isotretinoin.

2. Retin-A: Retin-A is a prescription cream that is applied to the skin to treat acne. The generic name for Retin-A is tretinoin.

3. Tetracycline: Tetracycline is an antibiotic taken orally to treat acne and respiratory infections.

Accutane

According to the Organization of Teratology Information Services (OTIS), approximately 25-35% of infants born to women exposed to Accutane during the first trimester of pregnancy showed a pattern of birth defects. This pattern includes craniofacial defects, heart defects, and central nervous system defects. There also is an increased risk of miscarriage and infant death associated with use of Accutane during pregnancy. It is safe to use Accutane when you are not pregnant and have discussed certain guidelines with your health care provider. If you are in your childbearing years you must use two forms of birth control, beginning one month prior to starting Accutane through one month after stopping Accutane. If you are breastfeeding you should not take Accutane. You must be counselled about the possible ways that your chosen birth control may fail. You must have a negative pregnancy test one week prior to taking Accutane. You must start Accutane on the 2nd or 3rd day after the next normal menstrual period.

Retin-A

According to OTIS, less than 10% of Retin-A passes into the mother's blood stream and less than that reaches the baby. Even with these findings, Retin-A still carries warnings of use by women who are pregnant or contemplating pregnancy. In this case it is best to discuss treatment with your dermatologist and other health care provider. Since not many studies have been done on Retin-A, it is best to avoid during pregnancy and follow the same guidelines as Accutane while consulting with your health care provider.

Tetracycline

According to OTIS, tetracycline appears to cause some inhibition of bone growth and discoloration of teeth in a fetus. Therefore, taking tetracycline should also be discussed with your dermatologist and other health care provider. Tetracycline should not be used during pregnancy unless recommended by your health care provider. The American Academy of Pediatrics has approved tetracycline safe for use during breastfeeding.

Conclusion

Despite what the major drug and pharmaceutical companies regularly suggest, it is now a pretty well established fact that not all chemically based commercial medical products are tested as thoroughly or extensively as they should be. For this reason, even though the manufacturers claim that they are 100% safe, there is good reason to suspect that the long term effects of using chemical based products may not be as well understood as you might think.

Chemical based products can also have unpleasant side effects, such as extremely dry skin, soreness, redness, irritation and excessive skin exfoliation. This happens because most chemical treatments work by counteracting the production of oil from the sebaceous glands, thus drying out the skin. This does reduce the severity of acne, but these side effects can be both unpleasant and painful.

That does not, however, suggest that you are entirely powerless in the fight against this debilitating condition. There are certainly things that can be done and changes that can be made that will either eliminate or reduce the severity of your acne during pregnancy.

1: The Acne Diet For Pregnant Women

One of the first things that you should consider when attempting to reduce or get rid of your acne is your diet, the things that you eat and drink every day. As the old cliché goes, you really are what you eat, and so if your diet is poor, then you cannot expect to be entirely healthy either. Your acne problem will certainly not be improved by a diet that is centered around the consumption of the wrong foodstuffs and liquids. Here is a list of dietary considerations that may help to alleviate your acne problems in an entirely natural and healthy manner:

Drink lots of water

Water is essential for healthy, supple and young looking skin, and has long been known to be one of the most effective treatments for any kind of adverse skin condition. This is partially because of its slightly alkaline nature (pH 7.3) and also the fact that it naturally prevents dehydration which can be a cause of the sebaceous glands over-producing oil and sebum. Basically, your skin needs plenty of water to function most efficiently and for this reason, most dermatologists and other skin care specialists recommend a minimum water intake of between six and eight glasses every day.

Cut out the wrong fats

Everyone knows that the average Western diet is far too rich in all the wrong types of fats and oils. With the prevalence of deep fried and 'fast' food, the average diet that a pregnant woman consumes is a natural aid to any acne problems that they may suffer. That is not to say that all fats are necessarily acne-friendly (as we will see) but those that contain trans-fatty acids such as milk and milk products, and margarine certainly are. In addition, artificially hydrogenated vegetable oils (most commonly used to cook fried and fats food) should be avoided, if possible.

While eating such fats does not necessarily cause acne, there is no doubt that the fats that are contained in such food items as ice cream, cheese, bacon and milk make the skin more prone to problems. The bottom line is that pimples and skin blemishes are at least partially caused by poor diet and improper hygiene, and consuming a diet that is rich in the wrong kind of fat and sugar is simply asking for trouble!

Polyunsaturated essential oils

These oils are called essential because that is exactly what they are – necessary for a long and healthy life. The two primary oils that women need are the

Omega-6 and Omega-3 oils, and, while the human body is in theory capable of producing them itself, it is relatively inefficient at doing so. For this reason, these need to be taken on board through your diet, and, as far as the health of your skin is concerned, it is the Omega-6 essential oils that are most important. Oil rich fish and fish-oil based food supplements like cod liver oil and other fish oils are the richest source of these essential oils. Even in the case of these essential oils, however, the current Western diet is not ideal, simply because the balance between Omega-6 and the Omega-3 is skewed.

Most experts agree that throughout human development, the balance between Omega-6 and 3 was approximately 2:1. However, the balance in the UK is now closer to 8:1, while in the USA it is 10:1 and in Australia it is closer to 12:1. Experts have no way of knowing at what point such imbalances will become harmful rather than beneficial, but there seems to be little doubt that at some point, that situation will manifest itself. So, eating a couple of portions of fatty fish like salmon every week will almost certainly help reduce acne related problems, principally because both of the Omega essential oils (present in salmon and other fish) are known to have marked anti-inflammatory qualities. If that is not possible, a daily dose of cod liver oil would be an effective alternative.

Raw vegetables

A skin friendly diet is one that emphasizes eating raw or lightly cooked vegetables, especially those of the leafy green variety that are rich in fibre as well as containing essential trace minerals. You should also include complex carbohydrates such as potatoes, pasta, rice and whole-grain bread because these also add additional fibre to your diet, which is important for keeping your system clean and free of accumulated toxins.

Try to eat three healthy meals a day and avoid snacking, as this is inevitably when you will turn to fatty or sugary foods. Foods that are rich in vitamin A such as broccoli and apricots will help keep acne at bay, as will lean red meat and whole grains, as they are rich in zinc. However, do not overdo the vitamin A, because your body will expel it extremely slowly, and too much in your body can be harmful.

Detoxifying

Like it or not, a fat laden diet is not good for your health in general, and will certainly not help you to deal with your acne problems. A healthy, balanced diet that is rich in the kind of foods highlighted above (especially raw vegetables) will, however, certainly help you. When you make the switch, however, be prepared for a few days of 'diet backlash' as your system gets used to the new regimen. You may find that you are noticeably more irritable than usual, and that you suffer bouts of nausea and headaches. That is your body purging itself of all the toxins and other harmful substances that you have accumulated as a result of your previously poor diet, so, once you have got over the first couple of days, the bad feelings will soon disappear. However, once your system is cleaned out in this way, and you switch to your new healthier diet, it is not only your acne problems that will decrease dramatically.

You will also find that you have far more energy than you ever had before and a marked improvement in mental clarity, so that you become a more effective and productive individual too. In addition, eating a diet that is based on raw and lightly cooked vegetables as well as plenty of fish helps to slow the aging process down, and should lead to a marked improvement in the general quality of both your skin and your life! And doing all of this just needs a simple change of diet – what could be more natural than that?

The vitamin B5 theory

There is no doubt that some vitamins, minerals and dietary supplements can help your fight against acne, although it is unlikely that any are going to enable you to 'cure' it completely! For example, as mentioned earlier, vitamin A can help your anti-acne fight, and zinc also appears to have a very positive effect. There are also some theories that acne is a result of a deficiency in vitamin B5, based on the idea that your body needs this to help metabolize the harmful fats in your diet.

The supporters of this theory suggest that in order to metabolize fats properly, your body needs Coenzyme-A, which is also necessary for the synthesis of hormones. Coenzyme-A is created within the body from a combination of cysteine, adenosine triphosphate, and vitamin B5 or pantothenic acid as it is otherwise known. Of these three, the one that is most commonly lacking is vitamin B5, and from this it follows that your body cannot make enough Coenzyme-A to satisfy all of its requirements.

In this case, the metabolization of fats takes precedence over the synthesis of hormones, and in this way, too many hormones remain unsynthesized. So, there is a need (according to this theory) for additional vitamin B5 to be taken in as a way of restoring the balance. The problem with this theory is that most proponents recommend extremely high dosages of B5 in order for the plan to be effective, with between 10 and 20 grams a day (note, that is grams, not milligrams) being the most widely recommended dose. There are many reports that, if taken in the dosages suggested, B5 is actually more harmful than beneficial.

For example, several (albeit non-scientific) studies have indicated that excessively large doses of B5 can lead to chronic fatigue, constant headaches and a general inability for the body to heal itself in the normal way. The proponents of the theory counter-claim that, since B5 is a water soluble vitamin, any unused excess will be secreted by the body, so there is no risk involved. While this is true to a certain extent, the fact is that the doses recommended by the supporters of the B5 theory are just too high for this to happen in reality. Your body simply does not have the capability of processing such massive amounts of any vitamin that quickly, and so the B5 will remain in your body long enough to cause the kind of problems that seem to be most commonly associated with it.

Most importantly, it is important to understand that everything that happens inside your body is about maintaining a healthy balance, and that the more balanced your system is, the more healthy you are. For example, your body needs both calcium and phosphorus to stay healthy, but it needs them in balance with one another. Get the balance wrong, and it is every bit as bad for you as not having them at all. Too much phosphorus, for example, and your body will start leeching calcium from your skeleton as a way of topping up your calcium store to maintain the correct balance between the two. This will obviously weaken your bones, making them far more susceptible to damage and breakages.

It is a similar story with vitamin B5. If you try to take in excessively high levels of any particular B vitamin, your body will react by attempting to leech all the other B vitamins out of your body to maintain the correct balance. So, your body 'sucks up' vitamins B3 and B6 from wherever it can find them, for example, and as these are key vitamins for controlling and regulating the levels of energy in your body, hence you get the feeling of being permanently tired. So, it appears that the vitamin B5 theory is simply not correct and that, if anything, taking vitamin B5 in the dosage that are most commonly recommended by the supporters of the theory is likely to be more dangerous than beneficial.

Acne and zinc

As suggested earlier, zinc is effective for countering the worst effects of acne, and that is perfectly true. However, that is not the full story, and there are other considerations that you need to be aware of. Zinc is extremely important to your body because it plays a critical role in more than 300 enzymatic reactions that take place naturally. It also is extremely important for the effective functioning of your immune system, because without the correct amounts of zinc in your system, several things can start to go wrong. For instance, your white blood cell count drops dramatically and the production of what are known as T-killer cells falls away drastically as well.

Both of these damage the immune system of your body, seriously reducing your ability to fight disease and sickness. That is why zinc can be used so effectively to reduce the duration and severity of several common sicknesses, including the common cold, as well as acne. In an ideal world, all of the zinc that you need would be taken in as part of your normal daily diet from such apparently zinc-rich foods as fish, red meat, legumes, egg yolks, soy products and whole grains.

However, modern farming methods have managed to dramatically reduce the amount of zinc that is actually present in most of these things nowadays. Zinc is a mineral that comes from the ground, and so for zinc to be present in your food, it must have been present in the ground where that food was grown (or, in the case of eggs and meat, in the feed that was given to the hens or the beef cattle). Modern farming methods (or more correctly, the fact that most land is over-farmed nowadays) mean that this is not the case, so it is less and less likely that you can get all of the zinc that you need to help fight your acne from your daily diet.

However, you should not be discouraged from trying zinc as part of your anti-acne diet, as it is one of the most effective tools against acne, and supplementing your diet with additional zinc is pretty cheap too. According to the majority of experts, the two types of zinc supplements that seem to be most effective in the battle against acne are Zinc gluconate and Zinc monomethionine (sometimes known as Opti-Zinc). Of these, most recommend the latter over the former, as it seems to be the most effective form of zinc when it comes to strengthening your immune system in the way that it needs, if it is to help in your fight.

You should also understand that there are such things as zinc inhibitors - other things that you take in that can drastically reduce the effectiveness of the zinc that you do ingest. For example, zinc and copper will fight against one another in your system for absorption in the gut, and copper almost always wins the fight! So, if there is excess copper in your body, it does not matter how much zinc you take in, it is not going to work. If you drink tap water that is delivered through copper pipes, then there will be trace elements of copper dumped into your system by every glass of water that you drink.

If, therefore, you are supplementing your diet with zinc and seeing no beneficial effects, it may well be that copper is winning the battle between the two minerals inside your body, so you should perhaps test for copper toxicity. The most accurate method for doing this is a 24-hour urine copper level test that can be carried out by your normal medical attendant. Testing for the levels of copper in your red blood cells may also work, but testing for copper levels in a hair sample is going to be far less reliable, because of the potential for external contamination.

If you can find someone who is skilled in a relatively unknown muscle testing process called applied kinesiology, they should also be capable of testing for excess levels of copper. In fact, this particular method of testing is something that you can learn to apply yourself, with a little practice, so it might be worth finding someone who can help you.

2: Tackling The Root Cause Of Pregnancy Acne

The idea behind all homeopathic medical treatments is that no condition can or should be viewed in isolation, and that curing people of anything is dependent on attacking the root cause of the problem at the source. It is all about treating the whole person, making them completely well in every way, rather than just attacking one medical condition on its own in the way that a normal medical attendant would. Furthermore, homeopathic treatment methods generally rely on encouraging the body to heal itself, rather than using invasive practices (such as surgery) or aggressive medicines and potions.

Adopting a homeopathic approach to the treatment of acne is therefore an extremely safe and effective treatment option. For this reason, it is easy to understand why there is growing popularity for homeopathic acne solutions. While this method of attacking acne enjoys variable levels of success – it works for some people, but not for others (usually those who are most severely affected) - this growing popularity is largely based on the fact that there are few or indeed no side effects.

Using homeopathic methods to treat acne is no more likely to generate immediate results than it is for any other medical condition. Homeopathy is a form of treatment that takes time to work, and there is no getting around that fact. The advantage of homeopathy, however, is that addresses all medical problems as symptoms rather than causes in themselves, and thus takes into account all aspects of an individual's health and general wellness before coming up with answers. This is as true of homeopathic treatment for acne as it is of any other condition, as acne treatment using homeopathic methods primarily focuses on the root cause of the condition rather than trying to treat the complaint at 'skin level'.

This is the reason why it is likely that a good homeopath may seem concerned about other aspects of your life that are apparently totally unconnected to your acne. They may, for example, ask about whether you suffer from stress as a part of your daily routine, and of course, as we have already established that your family history is an important contributory factor, they will most likely query you about that as well. They will most probably want to know about your life in general and all about the environment that you work, live or study in, before they decide on the best form of treatment for you.

They may prescribe some form of homeopathic medicine comprised of naturally occurring compounds such as:

Graphite

Silicea;

Hepar sulfuricum;

Calendula;

Kali brichomicum; or

Sulphur.

One point that you will often see raised by companies that make conventional drugs and medicines is that homeopathic medicines comprised of compounds and elements such as these have generally not been subjected to extensive clinical and scientific testing. And, while this is to a large extent true, it is a fact that certain homeopathic 'cures' do seem to have beneficial effects for many sufferers from acne without any adverse side effects. Homeopathy addresses acne as an outward sign or a manifestation that there is a deeper problem that needs dealing with. For that reason, you will never hear a homeopath prescribe ointments or creams, because this is only tackling the problem at the most superficial surface level, which is definitely not what homeopathy is all about.

The secret of homeopathy is that it adopts an entirely holistic approach, and views the whole person (the patient) both inside and out when they are seeking a cure or appropriate treatment for any condition that you have. It is all about discovering the root of your problems, rather than scratching at the surface. That is why it is extremely unlikely that a homeopath will treat what is, for you, a debilitating and scarring condition (both mentally and physically) as just another case of a few pimples!

So, taking advantage of the services of a homeopath is a great option for treating your acne, although you should accept that it is not going to be successful in every case. Nevertheless, because homeopathy targets the root cause of your acne, even if it does not cure it completely, it is extremely unlikely to do you any harm, and there is likely to be a complete lack of unpleasant side effects as well.

3: Bespoke Remedies For Pregnancy Acne

Ayurveda is an ancient Indian medical science which focuses on explaining hundreds of different diseases together with their symptoms and solutions based on what is known as Dosha theory. It also emphasizes the importance in the general 'wellness picture' of making lifestyle changes in response to illnesses and maladies.

Acne is defined as 'Youvana pitikas' in the terminology of Ayurvedic medicine, which literally translates as 'breakouts of youth'. And, while Ayurveda has a theory of why acne happens that is related to the youth of the sufferer, we are far more concerned with the solution or cures that it puts forward, rather than with the reasons that devotees of Ayurveda believe that acne occurs.

The fact is that Ayurvedic medicine suggests that healthy, strong skin not only protects the body, but beautifies it as well, and it is for the purposes of keeping the skin strong and healthy that Ayurveda proposes many solutions for acne. Some of these are herbal, while others are related to specific aspects of diet that are believed to contribute to the conditions that cause acne.

For example, it is believed that a combination of extracts from the following plants will form a highly effective treatment for acne and other conditions that might be associated with it:

Ikshu (Saccharumofficinarum);

Guduchi (Tinospora cardifolia);

Haritaki (Terminalia Chebula);

Lajjalu (Sensitive plant);

Gokshura (Tribulus terrestris L);

Kumari (Aloe Vera); and

Amalaki (Embelica officinalis).

And, when it comes to dietary considerations, it is believed that the following guidelines should be followed as well:

1. Consuming what Ayurveda considers to be 'opposite foods' at the same meal must be avoided. For instance, fish and milk are considered to be 'opposite' foods, as are pork and honey as well as milk and bananas.

2. Taking strenuous exercise followed by eating a heavy meal is to be avoided, as is eating heavy foods that might cause indigestion.

3. Excessive consumption of sour and salty foods, plus those that are relatively indigestible like radish or sesame is not good for your acne either, according to Ayurveda.

In addition, devotees of Ayurvedic medicine believe that there are additional steps that can be taken to lessen the severity of 'breakouts of youth'. These steps include:

1. Regularly massaging the face using herbal oils that contain Aloe Vera and gokshura;

2. Creating a face pack containing other beneficial herbs and applying it immediately after every massage.

It is widely claimed by the followers of Ayurveda that applying the regimen of massage followed by a natural herbal face pack for seven days will rid your skin of the pimples, pustules and lesions that are endemic to acne, and also removes dark circles around the eyes. The final belief of those that follow Ayurveda that you can use to help your acne relies on the fact that they believe that your emotions play a part in your acne problem as well. So, it is recommended that you learn to control your emotions and feelings using both meditation and yoga.

4: The Secrets Of Chinese Medicine

Before looking at the specific way that traditional Chinese medicine considers acne, it is probably worth looking in a little more detail at Chinese medicine and the theories behind it. Doing so will enable you to better understand exactly where the Chinese way of treating acne comes from.

The first thing to understand about traditional Chinese medicine is that it is primarily focused on treating or curing patients with natural herbal medicines and other techniques such as acupuncture. The theory is that there are two indispensable forces that affect the health and wellness of people, these being the Yin (female) and Yang (male). With reference to these two points of focus, all diseases, sicknesses and maladies are considered to be an external manifestation of an unhealthy imbalance between the two forces.

Therefore, it is the job of a doctor who practices traditional Chinese medicine to restore the necessary balance using medicines that are created from different traditional herbs and plant matter. Practitioners of traditional Chinese medicine further believe that there are they call the 'six external environmental forces' and that a imbalance between these is what causes most sicknesses and disease, including acne. These six environmental forces are:

1. Heat and summer heat;

2. Wind;

3. Cold;

4. Dryness;

5. Fire;

6. Dampness.

It is suggested that an imbalance between these six forces is what causes acne, and so different herbal remedies are recommended for different types of imbalances. The herbs that are used in traditional Chinese medicine are then divided into four herb 'groups', each of which is believed to have a specific bodily benefit. The particular benefits of each of these four herb 'groups' are:

1. Supplementing the strength, or strengthening the body;

2. Consolidating or redistributing qi (vitality or energy) as well as vital liquids such as blood around the body;

3. Dispersing or circulating qi and fluids, to relieve the accumulation of heat, cold, or dampness from various bodily organs;

4. Purging harmful waste matter from the body to relieve conditions caused by congestion in the body or an excess, and sometimes to eliminate toxins as well.

As far as acne is concerned, Chinese medicine usually considers it to be a result of the environmental force of heat and an excess build up of it inside the body of the acne sufferer. In other words, it is believed that too much heat in various parts of the body is directly responsible for the outbreak or acne. So, it follows that potions made from herbs that can dissipate what is considered to be an unhealthy build up of internal heat, at the same time as purging toxins from the body, are those that are usually given to acne sufferers.

Building a little further on the notion of acne being caused by heat inside the body, it is suggested by traditional Chinese herbalists that there are two different parts of the body where the heat forms that produce acne. These are:

1. Heat within the lungs;

2. Heat that builds up in the stomach and large intestine (known as Yang Ming).

It is believed that an excess of heat that is in the lungs pushes the toxins from that area of the body onto the skin surface, and it is build up of surface toxins that eventually causes acne. Alternatively, the second heat build up is in the stomach and intestine, caused by too much rich, fatty of spicy foods. This again generates toxins that are passed to the skin surface causing acne to break out as a direct result.

Chinese herbal acne 'recipes'

Many traditional Chinese doctors recommend the following three formulas for acne removal. In all three cases, combine the ingredients together and boil until all of the ingredients have been decocted:

Loquat leaf extract

15g Loquat leaf; 15g Dried rehmannia root; 15g Scrophularia root; 9g Mulberry bark; 9g Scutellaria root; 9g Coptis root; 9g Capejasmine fruit; 9g Red peony root; 9g Moutan bark; 9g Forsythia fruit; 9g Prunella spike; 9g White chrysanthemum flower.

Six drugs with additional ingredients

15g Honeysuckle flower; 15g Dandelion flower; 15g Chinese violet; 15g Chrysanthemum flower; 15g Forsythia fruit; 15g Dried rehmannia root; 9g Scutellaria root; 9g Moutan bark; 9g Tangerine seed; 9g Loquat leaf; 9g Platycodon root; 6g Licorice root.

Tangerines, oranges and safflower

9g Tangerine peel; 9g Pinellia tuber; 9g Poria; 9g Nutgrass flatsedge; 9g Zhejiang fritillaria bulb; 9g Orange kernel; 9g Safflower; 9g Red sage root; 9g Chinese angelica root; 9g Scutellaria root; 9g Forsythia fruit; 9g Loquat leaf; 6g Licorice root.

Garlic, lemons and potatoes

Although some people may find it hard to believe, there are many everyday items of foodstuff that can help with your acne in addition to those that you include in your new healthier diet. For example, one of the best home remedies that you can adapt to combat your acne is fresh garlic. All that needs to be done is to rub it four times a day on the areas of your skin that are most badly affected by your acne. Sure, it might not make you smell too good, but you are hardly likely to go out in public with garlic essence spread on your face, are you?

However, if you do this each and every day for a couple of weeks, then you are likely to see a significant improvement in the severity of the acne that you are suffering. In a similar manner, a combination of lemon juice and rose water can be very effective. Mix equal quantities of the two ingredients together and apply the mix to the infected areas. Leave the mix in place for around half an hour, and then simply wash it off using only warm water. Do this a few times a day for two weeks or so and you should start noticing that your acne will die down considerably. You can try to use lemon juice on its own to attack your acne in a slightly different way. You take the freshly squeezed lemon (or orange) juice and apply it to a cotton pad. Leave it on the affected skin areas for 20-30 minutes and then wash the juice off with warm water.

In all of these examples, the vitamins in the food stuff being applied to the acne affected area are good for your skin. They also dry the skin out, which helps to remove the sebum that is a necessary for the formation of the whiteheads, blackheads and lesions that are the bane of the life of every acne sufferer. Believe it or not, even the humble potato can help keep your acne problem at bay! Cut a raw potato in half and apply the flat, cut portion onto your skin. The potato is rich in vitamins, and these help to improve the overall condition of your skin. In addition, the alkaline nature of potatoes helps by breaking down the bacteria which have congregated in your pores, thus making it less likely that new acne blemishes will form later.

5: Herbal Antidotes For Pregnancy Acne

Not all natural herbal remedies are to be taken internally, although all of the Chinese medicines that we looked at earlier are. Another one that is taken by mouth is one which can help pre-empt the skin inflammation that is most commonly associated with acne. This is made up of equal proportions of herbal extracts taken from sarsaparilla, cleavers, yellow dock and burdock root.

These herbs are thought to be strong blood and lymph cleansing agents, and half a teaspoon of this blend three times every day should have a beneficial effect, especially when it is combined with a healthy diet such as that we looked at in a previous chapter. Other natural herbal treatments can be used as creams and potions that are applied to the affected areas of the skin as a way of reducing the acne-induced inflammation.

This is a particularly effective tactic when combined with the application of a warm compress to the skin beforehand, as this serves to open the skin pores, which gives the herbal remedy the best chance of working its healing powers on the affected skin area. We have already suggested that garlic, lemon juice and potatoes applied to the skin can help in reducing the worst effects of acne. There are a few more commonly used herbal acne remedies, although it should be noted that the effectiveness of using these treatments varies from person to person, and will depend to at least some extent on the severity of the acne that the sufferer has.

The worse the condition is, the more draconian and aggressive the method of treatment adopted is probably going to have to be. Using herbal remedies could never be described as aggressive, and so, while they all merit trying (there is nothing to lose, after all, as there are no side effects), there is no guarantee that they will work in any individual case. Red clover root can be applied to infected skin areas because it exhibits certain steroidal properties, which means that it is very effective for reducing swelling and inflammation. In a similar fashion, poke root and echinacea are sought after because of their anti-inflammatory characteristics, as are raw papaya and fresh mint.

All of these are effective antidotes to the inflammation and swellings caused by acne. Other combinations of herbs that can be externally applied to affected areas after the application of a warm compress which are known to work well for some people are:

Ground orange peel in water;

Nutmeg powder with fresh (unboiled) milk;

Ground ginger with milk;

Lemon juice with cinnamon;

Honey and cinnamon;

Boiled neem leaves;

Salt and vinegar; and

Turmeric and vinegar paste.

Herbs like chamomile, bergamot, juniper, dandelion root and witch hazel are all known to possess excellent astringent qualities too. This means that they can be applied to the skin with a little water in order to thoroughly clean the skin, thereby reducing the surface dirt and toxicity, which then improves the general condition of the sufferers skin in turn.

Herbal 'tea' paste

Combine the following ingredients together into a paste and apply to the infected areas of the skin:

2 parts Dandelion Root;

2 parts Red Clover;

1 part Alfalfa leaf;

1 part Echinacea root;

1/2 part Capsicum.

It is known to work wonders for some people, so give it a go, because there is nothing to lose by doing so – obviously there are no side-effects – and everything to potentially gain by doing so.

6: The Healing Power Of Green Tea

Across the world, the consumption of green tea is second only to water, and, over the past few years, the benefits of drinking it have become far more widely known, partially as a direct result of its ever increasing popularity. Several of the more prominent characteristics of green tea make it an ideal resource in your fight against the worst ravages of your acne. Originating from China (where the sheer size of the population is one of the reasons for its popularity) green tea is high in antioxidants, and these are famed for their ability to ward off diseases and keep the body's cell structure healthy.

Research has also indicated that antioxidants are an effective protection against cancer as well as being able to reduce the risk of heart disease and strokes. In some cases, they have even been known to reduce the levels of the 'bad' cholesterol blood levels in test subjects. In the past few years, however, it has become increasingly apparent that the antioxidant qualities of green tea may help to prevent or reduce the severity of acne as well. This may come as no great surprise, as it has long been suspected that placing a cold (or lukewarm) teabag on an acne blemish or lesion can help, by drawing out the toxins from the skin, thus promoting far faster healing times.

However, research into using green tea (from which most of the nutrients have not been removed) currently suggests that it can go much further than sticking a used teabag on your face. This research has indicated that green tea has an inherent ability to reduce swelling, redness and inflammation, fight bacteria and may even prevent excessive hormone activity as well. This is all very encouraging news for acne sufferers, as these are all present in the most severe cases of acne.

According to the results of tests that were reported to the American Academy of Dermatology, when a lotion is made up of 3% extract of green tea and applied to the skin, the test results were directly comparable to those seen using a commercial acne treatment cream that contained 4% benzoyl peroxide. In these tests (which were conducted using 100 test subjects over a period of twelve weeks) the cream that was made using green tea extract cream was seen to offer exactly the same level of effectiveness as a treatment for acne as benzoyl peroxide, but with far fewer unpleasant side effects.

While the latter is a common constituent of many leading brands of acne treatments, it is also used in the construction of tires and in plastic production as well as being a constituent of many proprietary brands of cosmetics. However, benzoyl peroxide is also known to be capable of irritating human skin, eyes and the respiratory tracts, and for this reason, it is even on the dangerous substance list of the Occupational Safety and Health Administration in the USA with a caution against the dangers of prolonged or long term exposure to it.

Of course, there are no such worries using green tea, as it is 100% natural, and has as yet no known side effects whatsoever. At the moment, it is widely believed that Western medical science is only scratching at the surface of all the medicinal benefits that using green tea might offer. One thing is for certain, however. If you want to avoid the irritation, the dry skin and unpleasant redness that often accompanies using commercial acne products based on benzoyl peroxide, there is now a safer but equally effective alternative in a cream or lotion made with green tea extract.

7: The Most Popular Natural Acne Remedies

Tea Tree Oil

Tea tree oil (which is often also referred to as melaleuca oil) is originally a native of Australia and can be completely clear to lightly gold-tinged in appearance. It is an oil that seems to have many natural acne fighting qualities, and because it is an entirely natural product, it has no nasty side effects either, hence its ever increasing popularity.

Licorice root extract

Licorice root and its extract has been used for medical purposes for thousands of years, with records showing that it may well have been used as far back as the Ancient Romans! While the earliest records indicate that it was usually used to settle upset stomachs (which is still its most common usage) it has nevertheless been shown to possess anti-inflammatory characteristics and qualities as well - hence its effectiveness in treating skin complaints like acne.

Olive leaf extract

In a similar fashion to the licorice root, the story of olive leaves and olive leaf extract as healers has a long history too, in this case being traceable all the way back to the ancient Greeks. Since that time, olive leaf extract has been used in many countries and societies as a medicinal herb, generally to ward off maladies such as coughs, colds, fevers and infections. This is often achieved through the consumption of olive leaf tea, but in addition, olive leaf extract has been used in many different ways to counter skin problems, including acne.

Aloe Vera extract

Aloe Vera extract is a widely used alternative to chemical based commercial acne creams, potions and ointments that has the major advantage of being far gentler and less aggressive, with no side effects. Aloe Vera extract contains some very effective anti-inflammatory agents and it can also help reduce the degree of scarring left by acne related lesions and blemishes.

Strawberry leaves

According to the scriptures of the Ancient Egyptians, they used wetted strawberry leaves applied to the infected areas as a way of treating a broad range of skin afflictions, including acne.

Basil tea

Drinking two or three cups of tea made with basil every day is an effective anti-bacterial agent that kills the germs that are one of the causes of acne from the inside. This is also effective against other forms of bacteria, so consuming tea infused with basil is always good for general health too.

Sandalwood

Sandalwood has long been recognized for its skin enhancing properties, so applying sandalwood oil to acne affected skin can return it to maximum health and vitality.

Burdock root

Crushed burdock root applied to affected areas of the skin is an effective way of treating many skin complaints, and it seems to be especially effective when used to combat acne.

8: How To Treat Other Skin Problems During Pregnancy

Pregnancy Mask

Among the most frustrating pregnancy skin problems is melasma, also known as chloasma or "pregnancy mask" - patches of dark, pigmented skin that appear on the face. Pregnancy mask is related to pregnancy hormones and sunlight exposure. The American Academy of Dermatology says women with darker complexions and dark hair are at greatest risk.

But regardless of your complexion, other areas of darker skin can also develop on or around your nipples and between your thighs. Many women also experience linea nigra or 'line of pregnancy', a darkened area of pigmentation that runs down the centre of the belly. While there is no specific treatment for pregnancy pigmentation problems, staying out of the sun can definitely diminish the amount of discoloration you experience, so can wearing a sunscreen anytime you are outdoors.

While the jury is still out on the safety of traditional skin-lightening ingredients such as hydroquinone during pregnancy, there are others with an established safety profile you can safely try. You can use azelaic acid, which is good for pigment, as well as any topical vitamin C product, which helps suppress pigment naturally. Phytocorrective Gel safely suppresses pigment, as well as the Aveeno soy-based products. They have a photo-stabilized sunscreen that contains soy and has been shown to lighten pigmented lesions on the skin.

If all else fails, you can safely cover pregnancy mask with a high-pigment concealer or foundation. For best results, choose the colour closest to your complexion and resist the urge to go lighter. If you select a light shade of concealer, you're not going to get better coverage, plus you're only going to draw attention to the mask by highlighting that area. Another tip is to always use a good moisturizer before putting on your concealer. This will help give better, more even coverage over large areas. If your mask does not clear after pregnancy, a chemical peel works like magic to remove all traces.

Pregnancy Belly Itches

From annoying belly itches to potentially serious body rashes, there is no question that pregnancy can sometimes make your skin crawl. Part of the problem is caused by hormones and part is the result of skin stretching, which also causes it to itch. Among the most common belly itches is PUPPP; short for pruritic urticarial papules and plaques of pregnancy. This is a hive-type reaction that commonly begins in the third trimester. It's first noticeable near the belly button, but it can quickly fan out over a wide area, including the thighs, breasts, and buttocks

While PUPPP isn't dangerous, and it often resolves soon after delivery, it can be incredibly uncomfortable.

If you just can't stand the itch, prescription-strength steroid creams can definitely help. You can also try dipping a cloth in some warm milk and applying it to the skin, or add a handful of oatmeal to a warm (not hot) bath. If your rash is itchy and contains fluid-filled blisters, talk to your doctor right away. This can be an autoimmune reaction known as pemphigoid gestationis or herpesgestationis. Although not related to the herpes virus, it can increase the risk of premature birth, and it may affect your baby's health as well, so it's vital to seek treatment early on.

Many women also suffer harmless, all-over itchiness during pregnancy. Often all that's needed to soothe the skin is calamine lotion or a good moisturizer. But again, bring any skin irritations to your doctor's attention. In rare instances, itchy skin can be a symptom of a pregnancy-related liver condition known as cholestasis, which may increase the risk of premature labor or cause some fetal distress.

Pregnancy Stretch Marks

From old-fashioned cocoa butter to high-tech skin creams that claim to prevent stretch marks, there is certainly no shortage of products to try. But today, most doctors believe that those red, blue, purple, and brown stretch marks that divide your belly like the Grand Canyon are largely hereditary, and most topical preparations won't prevent them from occurring.

But while you might not be able to prevent stretch marks, in many instances a few laser treatments after baby is born will cause your stretch marks to fade as quickly as your memory of labor pains. After the baby is born, treating stretch marks when they are red or purple can be accomplished with a pulse dye laser. Once they have turned beige, microdermabrasion, Retin A, Intense Pulsed Light and injections of fillers have varying degrees of success. If you want to try a topical preparation during pregnancy, glycolic acid creams or those containing green tea are most effective on stretch marks.

Pregnancy, Botox, and Wrinkle Fillers

Finally, in case you're wondering whether or not it's safe to get anti-ageing wrinkle treatments like Botox or Restylane during pregnancy, it's important to note that there have been no tests to confirm safety. However, many women have had wrinkle injections and then got pregnant within a couple of months and went on to deliver perfect, healthy babies.

www.ingramcontent.com/pod-product-compliance
Lightning Source LLC
Chambersburg PA
CBHW070838290526
45795CB00002B/900